THE ULTIMATE ATKINS DIET COOKBOOK FOR BEGINNERS

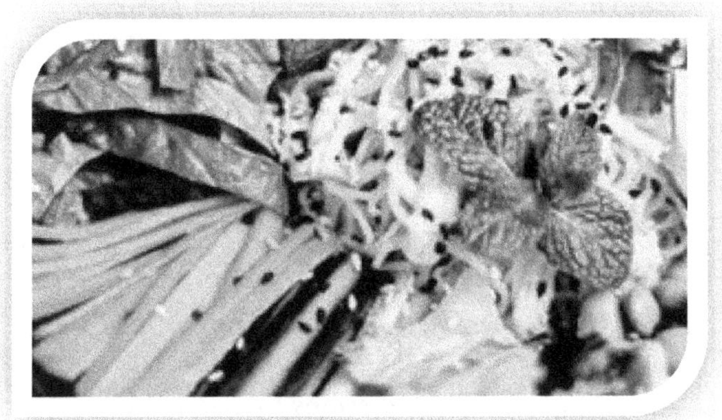

Quick and Easy, Delicious Low-Carb Recipes with a 30-Day Meal Plan for Weight Loss and Healthy Eating.

Dr. Linda B. Allen

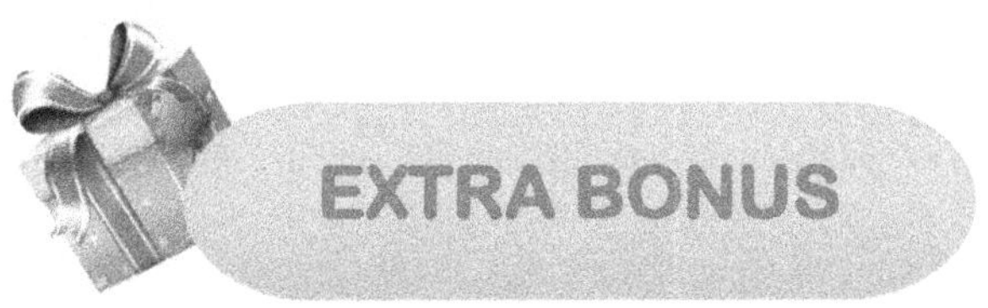

BONUS NO. 1

WEEKLY MEAL PLANNER

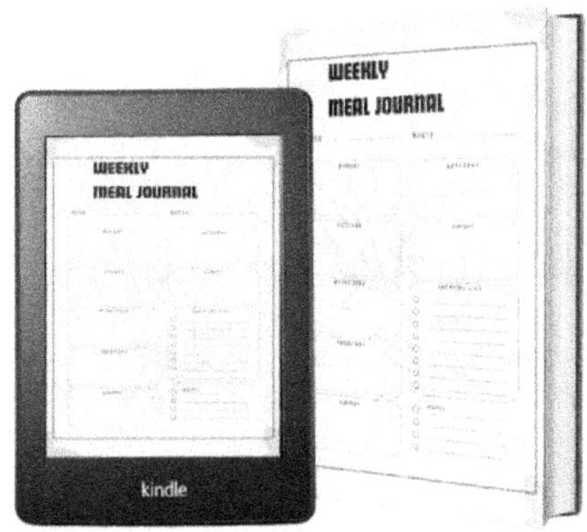

BONUS N0: 2

ENHANCING SUCCESS ON THE ATKINS DIET

SCAN THE QR-CODE BELOW FOR MORE BOOKS FROM THIS AUTHOR

TABLE OF CONTENTS

Greetings, fellow seekers of health and vitality,

Within the pages of this cookbook lies a journey, a journey toward holistic wellness, a path where the amalgamation of flavorful recipes, evidence-based nutritional guidance, and pragmatic meal planning converges. As a doctor specializing in nutrition and diet, I've had the privilege of accompanying numerous individuals on their quests for healthier lives. This book, "The Ultimate Atkins Diet Cookbook for Beginners," embodies the culmination of years of expertise, passion, and a relentless pursuit of helping others achieve their health goals.

In today's ever-evolving world, the pursuit of well-being has become a universal endeavor. Amid the cacophony of dietary trends and wellness philosophies, the Atkins Diet has stood as a steadfast beacon, guiding individuals toward sustainable weight loss and improved health. This book is not just a compilation of recipes; it's a doorway into a transformative lifestyle, crafted to empower, educate, and inspire.

The Atkins Diet isn't just a fleeting fad; it's a scientifically-backed methodology designed to reshape one's relationship with food and harness the body's natural ability to burn fat for fuel. In these chapters, we'll unravel the intricacies of the Atkins Diet, elucidating its phases, debunking myths, and underscoring the scientific rationale behind its efficacy. It's not just about shedding pounds; it's about fostering a sustainable and balanced approach to eating.

At the heart of this book lies a treasure trove of tantalizing recipes meticulously curated to tantalize taste buds while adhering to the principles of the Atkins Diet. From sunrise to sunset, from hearty breakfasts to satiating dinners, every recipe is a celebration of flavors and textures, carefully crafted to ensure that healthy eating is not just a choice but a delight.

The 30-day meal plan encapsulated within these pages isn't merely a list of meals; it's a comprehensive roadmap. Each day's plan is intricately designed, considering nutritional balance, variety, and simplicity. It's a blueprint for success, guiding readers through each phase of the Atkins Diet, providing shopping lists and correlated recipes, all aimed at making the journey seamless and enjoyable.

However, this book isn't confined to the kitchen. It's a holistic guide, addressing exercise regimens, dispelling common myths, and providing tools to surmount obstacles on the path to better health. Empowerment through knowledge is our ethos, and every chapter is imbued with evidence-based information to guide readers toward informed choices.

"The Ultimate Atkins Diet Cookbook for Beginners" isn't just another addition to your cookbook collection; it's a promise, a promise of transformation, of renewed vitality, and a greater comprehension of the profound relationship between nutrition and health.

My dedication to guiding individuals toward healthier lifestyles echoes through these pages. This book is more than a compilation; it's a testament to my commitment to fostering lasting change, one plate at a time.

Join me on this journey, where health, flavor, and knowledge intertwine to create a symphony of well-being.

With warm regards and a passion for good health,

[Dr. Linda B. Allen]

Understanding the Atkins Diet:

In the landscape of diets and weight management strategies, the Atkins Diet has emerged as a paradigm shift in nutritional philosophy. Founded by Dr. Robert Atkins, this approach challenges the conventional belief that fat is the enemy and champions the use of the body's innate ability to burn fat as fuel. At its core, the Atkins Diet is a low-carbohydrate eating plan that emphasizes protein and healthy fats while limiting refined carbohydrates.

Principles and Phases of the Atkins Diet:

The Atkins Diet operates on the premise that by reducing carbohydrate intake, the body transitions into a state of ketosis, where it primarily burns fat for energy. This diet is structured into four distinct phases:

Induction Phase: The inaugural phase jumpstarts the body into ketosis by significantly restricting carbohydrates (typically less than 20 grams per day). During this phase, the emphasis is on high-fat, high-protein foods to kickstart fat burning.

Balancing Phase (OWL - Ongoing Weight Loss): Gradually, more nuts, low-carb vegetables, and small portions of fruits are introduced to the diet to determine an individual's critical carbohydrate threshold for continued weight loss without gaining.

Fine-Tuning Phase (Pre-Maintenance): As one approaches their weight loss goal, this phase focuses on fine-tuning the diet by slowly adding more carbohydrates while monitoring weight loss and ensuring it remains steady.

Maintenance Phase: At this stage, the diet becomes a sustainable lifestyle. Carbohydrate intake can be increased further as long as weight maintenance is maintained. Healthy eating becomes second nature, emphasizing whole, unprocessed foods.

Benefits of Low-Carb Eating for Weight Loss:

The Atkins Diet boasts an array of benefits, with weight loss being a primary advantage. By minimizing refined carbohydrates, blood sugar levels stabilize, reducing cravings and fluctuations in energy levels.

Furthermore, the diet often leads to a decrease in triglycerides, an increase in HDL (good) cholesterol, and improved markers for heart health. Low-carb diets like Atkins have also shown promise in managing conditions like type 2 diabetes and metabolic syndrome.

Getting Started with the Atkins Diet:

Embarking on the Atkins Diet necessitates a fundamental shift in dietary habits. Before commencing, it's crucial to understand the fundamentals and arm oneself with the right tools:

Educate Yourself: Understanding the science behind the diet, its phases, and the role of carbohydrates, proteins, and fats is crucial. Resources like books, reputable websites, or seeking guidance from a healthcare professional versed in the Atkins Diet can be immensely beneficial.

Plan Your Meals: Planning is pivotal. Design meal plans that align with the diet's principles, ensuring they're diverse, satisfying, and within the recommended carbohydrate limits for each phase.

Stock Your Pantry: A well-stocked kitchen is essential. Ensure you have a variety of low-carb foods, such as lean meats, fish, eggs, low-carb vegetables, nuts, seeds, and healthy fats like olive oil and avocados.

Monitor Progress: Keeping track of food intake, weight, energy levels, and how your body responds to the diet is invaluable. This can be achieved through food journals, tracking apps, or regular check-ins with a nutritionist or dietitian.

Essential Guidelines and Tools:

The Atkins Diet isn't just about restricting carbohydrates; it's about making informed dietary choices. Here are some essential guidelines and tools to aid your Atkins journey:

Carbohydrate Counting: Understanding the carbohydrate content in foods is crucial. Familiarize yourself with the carbohydrate counts of common foods to stay within the recommended limits for each phase.

Net Carbs: In the Atkins Diet, net carbs are calculated by subtracting fiber and sugar alcohols from the total carbohydrates. This is a key factor in determining the impact of carbs on blood sugar levels.

Reading Labels: Learning to read nutrition labels can help in identifying hidden sugars and carbohydrates in packaged foods. Look out for ingredients like maltitol, sorbitol, and other sugar alcohols.

Support and Community: Joining support groups or online communities can provide invaluable encouragement, tips, and motivation, making the Atkins journey more enjoyable and sustainable.

Consultation: It's advisable, especially for those with pre-existing health conditions, to consult with a healthcare professional or a registered dietitian before embarking on the Atkins Diet. This ensures personalized guidance and addresses any concerns or potential risks.

The Atkins Diet isn't a one-size-fits-all solution, but for many, it has proven to be an effective means of weight management and improving overall health. Understanding its principles, embracing its phases, and adhering to essential guidelines while utilizing the right tools can pave the way for a successful Atkins journey, leading to improved health and vitality.

What is the Atkins Diet?

At its core, the Atkins Diet is a low-carbohydrate, high-protein eating plan designed to shift the body's metabolism from using glucose as its primary fuel source to utilizing stored fat for energy. It focuses on the body's natural ability to enter a state of ketosis, wherein fat becomes the primary energy source, resulting in weight loss and other health improvements.

How the Atkins Diet Works: Four Phases Explained:

The Atkins Diet operates through four distinctive phases, each serving a specific purpose in facilitating weight loss and transitioning to a sustainable low-carb lifestyle:

Induction Phase: This phase jumpstarts the diet by restricting carbohydrate intake to 20-25 grams per day for two weeks. High-fat, high-protein foods like meats, fish, eggs, and low-carb vegetables are emphasized to trigger ketosis, kickstarting rapid weight loss.

Balancing Phase (OWL - Ongoing Weight Loss): Gradually, more nuts, seeds, low-carb vegetables, and small portions of fruits are introduced. This phase aims to find an individual's critical carbohydrate intake level for continued weight loss without regaining.

Fine-Tuning Phase (Pre-Maintenance): As the weight loss goal approaches, the focus shifts to fine-tuning the diet by slowly adding more carbohydrates while ensuring steady weight loss.

Maintenance Phase: At this stage, individuals have reached their desired weight and transition into a lifelong maintenance plan. Carbohydrate intake is increased further, focusing on healthy choices while maintaining weight and overall health.

Foods to Embrace and Avoid in the Atkins Diet:

The Atkins Diet encourages specific foods while limiting or avoiding others to maintain low-carbohydrate intake:

Foods to Embrace:

Proteins: Meats (chicken, beef, pork), fish, eggs, tofu, and other sources of lean protein.

Healthy Fats: Olive oil, avocados, nuts, seeds, and fatty fish like salmon are encouraged.

Low-Carb Vegetables: Leafy greens, broccoli, cauliflower, zucchini, and bell peppers are staples due to their low carbohydrate content.

Foods to Avoid or Limit:

High-Carb Foods: Refined sugars, grains, starchy vegetables (like potatoes and corn), and most fruits high in sugar content.

Processed Foods: Packaged foods high in refined carbohydrates, trans fats, and added sugars should be minimized or avoided.

Sugary Beverages: Soda, fruit juices, and sugary drinks are discouraged due to their high sugar content.

Benefits of Low-Carb Eating for Weight Loss:

The Atkins Diet and other low-carb approaches offer a multitude of benefits beyond weight loss:

Effective Weight Loss: The reduction in carbohydrates leads to decreased insulin levels, promoting fat burning and weight loss.

Stable Blood Sugar: Low-carb diets help regulate blood sugar levels, making them beneficial for individuals with diabetes or insulin resistance.

Improved Heart Health: Lowering carb intake often leads to improved cholesterol levels, decreased triglycerides, and increased HDL (good) cholesterol.

Reduced Cravings and Hunger: Protein and fats promote satiety, reducing cravings and feelings of hunger, aiding in adherence to the diet.

Common Myths and Misconceptions:

Despite the numerous benefits supported by research, low-carb diets like Atkins often face misconceptions and myths:

Myth: Low-Carb Diets are Unhealthy: Contrary to popular belief, well-formulated low-carb diets emphasize healthy fats, lean proteins, and nutrient-rich vegetables, supporting overall health.

Myth: Low-Carb Diets Lead to Nutrient Deficiencies: When planned thoughtfully, low-carb diets can provide adequate nutrients through a variety of foods, ensuring a well-rounded intake.

Myth: Low-Carb Diets are Unsustainable: With proper guidance and understanding, low-carb diets can be sustainable long-term lifestyles, promoting weight maintenance and overall health.

In essence, the Atkins Diet embodies a strategic low-carbohydrate approach to weight loss and improved health.

SIt aims to reset the body's metabolism, transitioning it from a reliance on carbohydrates to a state of utilizing stored fat for energy. By understanding its principles, embracing the recommended foods, and dispelling common misconceptions, individuals can harness the potential benefits of a low-carb lifestyle, paving the way for sustainable weight loss and improved well-being.

Breakfast Recipes: Low-Carb and High-Energy Starters:

1. Spinach and Feta Omelette

Ingredients:

- 2 large eggs
- 1 cup fresh spinach, chopped
- 1/4 cup crumbled feta cheese
- 1 tablespoon olive oil
- Salt and pepper to taste

Preparation:

1. Beat the eggs and add salt and pepper to taste in a bowl.
2. Heat olive oil in a non-stick skillet over medium heat.
3. Add the chopped spinach to the skillet and cook until wilted.
4. Pour the beaten eggs over the spinach and swirl the pan to spread evenly.
5. Once the edges set, sprinkle the feta cheese over half of the omelette and fold it in half.
6. Cook until the cheese melts, about 1 more minute.
7. Serve hot with a side of avocado or tomatoes.

Portion Size: One serving

Nutritional Information: Approximately 280 calories, 20g fat, 4g carbohydrates, 19g protein

2. Greek Yogurt Parfait

Ingredients:

- 1/2 cup full-fat Greek yogurt
- 1/4 cup of fresh berries, such as blueberries and strawberries
- 1 tablespoon chopped nuts (e.g., almonds, walnuts)
- 1 teaspoon chia seeds (optional)
- Stevia or a drizzle of sugar-free syrup (optional)

Preparation:

1. In a glass or bowl, layer the Greek yogurt, fresh berries, and chopped nuts.
2. Optionally, add a sprinkle of chia seeds for extra fiber.
3. Sweeten with stevia or a drizzle of sugar-free syrup, if desired.
4. Serve chilled.

Portion Size: One serving

Nutritional Information: Approximately 200 calories, 12g fat, 10g carbohydrates, 15g protein

3. Avocado and Bacon Breakfast Bowl

Ingredients:

- 1 ripe avocado, halved and pitted
- 2 strips of bacon, cooked and chopped
- 2 eggs, cooked to preference (fried, scrambled)
- Salt and pepper to taste

Preparation:

1. Scoop out a portion of the avocado to create a bowl-like cavity.
2. Fill the avocado halves with cooked eggs.
3. Top with chopped bacon.
4. Season with salt and pepper to taste.
5. Serve immediately.

Portion Size: One serving

Nutritional Information: Approximately 350 calories, 28g fat, 9g carbohydrates, 17g protein

4. Coconut Flour Pancakes

Ingredients:

- 2 tablespoons coconut flour
- 2 eggs
- 1/4 teaspoon baking powder
- 1 tablespoon coconut oil (for cooking)
- Sugar-free syrup or berries for topping (optional)

Preparation:

1. In a bowl, whisk together the coconut flour, eggs, and baking powder until well combined.
2. Heat coconut oil in a non-stick skillet over medium heat.
3. Spoon small portions of the batter onto the skillet to form pancakes.
4. Cook for 2-3 minutes on each side until golden brown.
5. Serve hot with sugar-free syrup or fresh berries, if desired.

Portion Size: 2-3 pancakes (depending on size)

Nutritional Information: Approximately 250 calories, 18g fat, 8g carbohydrates, 10g protein

5. Smoked Salmon and Cream Cheese Roll-ups

Ingredients:

- 4 slices of smoked salmon
- 2 tablespoons cream cheese
- 1 tablespoon chopped chives or dill
- Thinly sliced cucumber or avocado (optional)

Preparation:

1. Lay out the smoked salmon slices on a clean surface.
2. Spread a thin layer of cream cheese over each slice.
3. Sprinkle chopped chives or dill evenly over the cream cheese.
4. Optionally, add thinly sliced cucumber or avocado.
5. Roll up the salmon slices and secure with toothpicks if needed.
6. Serve chilled.

Portion Size: One serving

Nutritional Information: Approximately 180 calories, 12g fat, 2g carbohydrates, 15g protein

Ingredients:

- 4 large eggs
- 1 cup shredded zucchini
- 1/2 cup shredded cheddar cheese
- Salt, pepper, and herbs of choice (e.g., parsley, thyme)

Preparation:

1. Preheat the oven to 350°F (175°C) and grease a muffin tin.
2. In a bowl, beat the eggs and season with salt, pepper, and herbs.
3. Stir in the shredded zucchini and cheddar cheese.
4. Pour the mixture into the prepared muffin tin, filling each cup about 3/4 full.
5. Bake for 15-20 minutes until the muffins are set and slightly golden.
6. Before serving, allow them to cool slightly.

Portion Size: Two muffins per serving

Nutritional Information: Approximately 220 calories, 16g fat, 4g carbohydrates, 15g protein

7. Cauliflower Hash Browns

Ingredients:

- 2 cups grated cauliflower
- 1 egg
- 1/4 cup grated parmesan cheese
- 1/4 teaspoon garlic powder
- Salt and pepper to taste
- Cooking oil for frying

Preparation:

1. Squeeze excess moisture out of the grated cauliflower using a clean kitchen towel.
2. In a bowl, combine the cauliflower, egg, parmesan cheese, garlic powder, salt, and pepper.
3. In a skillet over medium heat, preheat cooking oil.
4. Form small patties from the cauliflower mixture and place them in the skillet.
5. Cook for 3-4 minutes on each side until golden brown.

6. Drain on paper towels before serving.

Portion Size: One serving (2-3 hash browns)

Nutritional Information: Approximately 180 calories, 12g fat, 8g carbohydrates, 10g protein

8. Turkey and Cheese Breakfast Roll-ups

Ingredients:

4 slices deli turkey or chicken slices

2 slices cheese (cheddar, Swiss, or your choice)

1 tablespoon mustard or mayonnaise

Lettuce leaves or spinach (optional)

Preparation:

1. Lay out the turkey or chicken slices on a flat surface.
2. Spread mustard or mayonnaise evenly over each slice.
3. Place a slice of cheese on top of each slice.
4. Optionally, add lettuce leaves or spinach.
5. Roll up the slices and secure with toothpicks if needed.
6. Serve chilled or at room temperature.

Portion Size: One serving

Nutritional Information: Approximately 220 calories, 15g fat, 2g carbohydrates, 18g protein

9. Chia Seed Pudding

Ingredients:

- 2 tablespoons chia seeds
- Half a cup of almond milk, unsweetened (or any other preferred milk)
- 1/4 teaspoon vanilla extract
- Stevia or sugar-free sweetener (optional)
- Berries or nuts for topping (optional)

Preparation:

1. In a bowl or jar, mix chia seeds, almond milk, vanilla extract, and sweetener (if using).
2. Stir well to combine and let it sit for 10 minutes.
3. Stir again to prevent clumping and refrigerate overnight or for at least 2 hours until it thickens.
4. Top with berries or nuts before serving, if desired.

Portion Size: One serving

Nutritional Information: Approximately 150 calories, 9g fat, 10g carbohydrates, 5g protein

10. Keto Green Smoothie

Ingredients:

1 cup unsweetened almond milk

- 1/2 ripe avocado
- 1/2 cup spinach or kale leaves
- 1/4 cup cucumber chunks
- 1/4 cup frozen berries (optional)
- 1 tablespoon chia seeds or flaxseeds
- Stevia or sugar-free sweetener (optional)

Preparation:

1. Blend all the ingredients until smooth and creamy.
2. Add sweetener if desired for extra sweetness.
3. Serve chilled.

Portion Size: One serving

Nutritional Information: Approximately 200 calories, 16g fat, 10g carbohydrates, 5g protein

Lunch Recipes: Satisfying and Quick Low-Carb Meals:

1. Grilled Chicken Caesar Salad

Ingredients:

- 4 oz grilled chicken breast
- 2 cups romaine lettuce, chopped
- 1 tablespoon grated Parmesan cheese
- 2 tablespoons Caesar dressing (low-carb)
- Salt, pepper, and garlic powder to taste
- Optional: cherry tomatoes, cucumber slices

Preparation:

1. Season the grilled chicken breast with salt, pepper, and garlic powder.
2. Grill the chicken until fully cooked and let it rest before slicing.
3. In a bowl, toss chopped romaine lettuce with Caesar dressing.
4. Top the salad with sliced grilled chicken, grated Parmesan, and additional veggies if desired.

Portion Size: One serving

Nutritional Information: Approximately 250 calories, 10g fat, 4g carbohydrates, 30g protein

Ingredients:

- 2 medium zucchinis (spiralized into noodles)
- 2 tablespoons pesto sauce (low-carb)
- 1/2 cup cherry tomatoes, halved
- 1 tablespoon olive oil
- To taste, add crushed red pepper flakes, salt, and pepper.
- Optional: grated Parmesan cheese

Preparation:

1. Heat olive oil in a skillet over medium heat.
2. Add zucchini noodles and cherry tomatoes to the skillet.
3. Sauté for 3-4 minutes until the noodles are tender.
4. Stir in pesto sauce and season with salt, pepper, and red pepper flakes.
5. Cook for an additional minute.
6. Serve hot with optional grated Parmesan cheese on top.

Portion Size: One serving

Nutritional Information: Approximately 200 calories, 15g fat, 8g carbohydrates, 5g protein

3. Turkey Lettuce Wraps

Ingredients:

- 4 large lettuce leaves (butter lettuce or romaine)
- 4 oz sliced turkey breast
- 1/2 avocado, sliced
- 1/4 cup shredded carrots
- 1/4 cup sliced cucumbers
- 2 tablespoons hummus (low-carb)
- Optional: chopped bell peppers, cherry tomatoes

Preparation:

1. Lay out the lettuce leaves on a flat surface.
2. Spread hummus on each lettuce leaf.
3. Layer with sliced turkey, avocado, shredded carrots, and cucumbers.
4. Add additional veggies if desired.
5. Roll up the lettuce leaves like a wrap and secure with toothpicks if needed.

Portion Size: One serving (2 lettuce wraps)

Nutritional Information: Approximately 220 calories, 10g fat, 10g carbohydrates, 20g protein

4. Cauliflower Fried Rice with Shrimp

Ingredients:

- 2 cups cauliflower rice
- 6 oz cooked shrimp
- 1/4 cup diced bell peppers
- 1/4 cup diced onions
- 1/4 cup peas (optional or in moderation)
- 2 tablespoons soy sauce (or tamari for low-carb)
- 1 tablespoon sesame oil
- 2 eggs, beaten
- Salt, pepper, and garlic powder to taste

Preparation:

1. Heat sesame oil in a large skillet or wok over medium heat.
2. Add diced bell peppers and onions, and sauté until softened.
3. Stir in cauliflower rice and peas, if using, and cook for 3-4 minutes.

4. Push the rice mixture to one side of the skillet and pour the beaten eggs into the other side.

5. Scramble the eggs until cooked and mix with the rice.

6. Add cooked shrimp and soy sauce to the skillet, and season with salt, pepper, and garlic powder.

7. Stir-fry for an additional 2-3 minutes.

8. Serve hot.

Portion Size: One serving

Nutritional Information: Approximately 250 calories, 10g fat, 12g carbohydrates, 25g protein

5. Greek Salad with Grilled Halloumi

Ingredients:

- 2 cups mixed greens (lettuce, spinach)
- 3 oz grilled halloumi cheese, sliced
- 1/4 cup cherry tomatoes, halved
- 2 tablespoons sliced Kalamata olives
- 1/4 cup diced cucumbers
- 2 tablespoons Greek dressing (low-carb)
- Optional: fresh herbs (oregano, parsley)

Preparation:

1. Arrange mixed greens on a plate.
2. Top with grilled halloumi slices, cherry tomatoes, Kalamata olives, and diced cucumbers.
3. Drizzle Greek dressing over the salad and garnish with fresh herbs if desired.

Portion Size: One serving

Nutritional Information: Approximately 300 calories, 20g fat, 8g carbohydrates, 15g protein

6. Egg Salad Lettuce Wraps

Ingredients:

- 4 large lettuce leaves (butter lettuce or romaine)
- 4 hard-boiled eggs, chopped
- 2 tablespoons mayonnaise (or Greek yogurt for a lighter option)
- 1 tablespoon Dijon mustard
- 1/4 cup diced celery
- Salt, pepper, and paprika to taste
- Optional: chopped green onions

Preparation:

1. In a bowl, mix chopped hard-boiled eggs, mayonnaise, Dijon mustard, diced celery, salt, pepper, and paprika.
2. Spoon the egg salad onto each lettuce leaf.
3. Garnish with chopped green onions if desired.
4. Wrap the lettuce around the egg salad and serve.

Portion Size: One serving (2 lettuce wraps)

Nutritional Information: Approximately 220 calories, 18g fat, 3g carbohydrates, 12g protein

7. Low-Carb Turkey Taco Lettuce Cups

Ingredients:

- 4 large lettuce leaves (iceberg or Boston lettuce)
- 4 oz cooked ground turkey (seasoned with taco seasoning)
- 1/4 cup diced tomatoes
- 2 tablespoons diced onions
- 2 tablespoons shredded cheese (cheddar or Mexican blend)
- 2 tablespoons sour cream (optional)
- Fresh cilantro for garnish (optional)

Preparation:

1. Divide cooked ground turkey evenly among lettuce leaves.
2. Top each lettuce cup with diced tomatoes, onions, shredded cheese, and sour cream if using.
3. Garnish with fresh cilantro if desired and serve.

Portion Size: One serving (2 lettuce cups)

Nutritional Information: Approximately 250 calories, 15g fat, 6g carbohydrates, 20g protein

8. Chicken and Avocado Salad

Ingredients:

- 4 oz grilled chicken breast, sliced
- 1/2 avocado, sliced
- 2 cups mixed greens (lettuce, spinach)
- 1/4 cup sliced cucumbers
- 1/4 cup sliced radishes
- 2 tablespoons vinaigrette dressing (low-carb)
- Salt, pepper, and herbs to taste

Preparation:

1. Arrange mixed greens on a plate.
2. Top with sliced grilled chicken, avocado, cucumbers, and radishes.
3. Drizzle vinaigrette dressing over the salad and season with salt, pepper, and herbs.

Portion Size: One serving

Nutritional Information: Approximately 280 calories, 15g fat, 8g carbohydrates, 25g protein

9. Tuna Stuffed Bell Peppers

Ingredients:

- 2 bell peppers, halved and seeds removed
- 1 can (5 oz) tuna, drained
- 1/4 cup diced celery
- 2 tablespoons mayonnaise (or Greek yogurt)
- 1 tablespoon chopped pickles
- Salt, pepper, and paprika to taste
- Optional: shredded cheese for topping

Preparation:

1. Preheat the oven to 375°F (190°C).
2. In a bowl, mix drained tuna, diced celery, mayonnaise, chopped pickles, salt, pepper, and paprika.
3. Stuff each bell pepper half with the tuna mixture.
4. Optionally, sprinkle shredded cheese on top.
5. Place the stuffed peppers on a baking sheet and bake for 20-25 minutes until peppers are tender.

Portion Size: One serving (2 pepper halves)

Nutritional Information: Approximately 220 calories, 12g fat, 10g carbohydrates, 20g protein

10. Keto Chicken Cobb Salad

Ingredients:

- 4 oz grilled chicken breast, sliced
- 2 cups mixed greens (lettuce, spinach)
- 2 slices cooked bacon, crumbled
- 1 hard-boiled egg, sliced
- 1/4 cup diced tomatoes
- 1/4 cup diced cucumbers

- 2 tablespoons blue cheese crumbles

- 2 tablespoons ranch dressing (low-carb)

- Salt, pepper, and herbs to taste

Preparation:

1. Arrange mixed greens on a plate.

2. Top with sliced grilled chicken, crumbled bacon, sliced egg, tomatoes, cucumbers, and blue cheese.

3. Drizzle ranch dressing over the salad and season with salt, pepper, and herbs.

Portion Size: One serving

Nutritional Information: Approximately 320 calories, 20g fat, 8g carbohydrates, 25g protein

Dinner Recipes: Flavorful Low-Carb Dishes:

1. Lemon Garlic Butter Salmon

Ingredients:

- 4 salmon fillets (4-6 oz each)
- 2 tablespoons melted butter
- 2 cloves garlic, minced
- 1 lemon (zest and juice)
- Garnish with Salt, pepper, and fresh parsley

Preparation:

1. Preheat oven to 375°F (190°C) and line a baking sheet with parchment paper.
2. Arrange the salmon fillets onto the baking sheet that has been prepared.
3. In a bowl, mix melted butter, minced garlic, lemon zest, and lemon juice.
4. Brush the butter mixture over each salmon fillet.
5. Season with salt and pepper.
6. Bake the salmon for 12-15 minutes, or until its thoroughly done.
7. Garnish with fresh parsley before serving.

Portion Size: One serving

Nutritional Information: Approximately 300 calories, 20g fat, 2g carbohydrates, 30g protein

2. Cauliflower Crust Pizza

Ingredients:

- 1 head cauliflower, grated (about 3 cups)
- 1 egg
- 1/2 cup shredded mozzarella cheese
- 1/4 cup grated Parmesan cheese
- 1 teaspoon Italian seasoning
- Pizza sauce, shredded cheese, and desired toppings

Preparation:

1. Preheat oven to 400°F (200°C).
2. Place grated cauliflower in a microwave-safe bowl and microwave for 5 minutes.
3. Let it cool, then squeeze out excess moisture using a clean kitchen towel.
4. In a bowl, mix cauliflower, egg, mozzarella, Parmesan, and Italian seasoning.

5. Spread the mixture on a lined baking sheet to form a crust.

6. Bake the crust for 15-20 minutes, or until brown.

7. Add pizza sauce, shredded cheese, and desired toppings.

8. Bake for an additional 10-15 minutes until the cheese melts and toppings are cooked.

Portion Size: One-fourth of the pizza

Nutritional Information: Approximately 250 calories, 15g fat, 10g carbohydrates, 15g protein

3. Grilled Lemon Herb Chicken

Ingredients:

- 4 boneless, skinless chicken breasts
- 2 tablespoons olive oil
- 2 cloves garlic, minced
- Zest and juice of 1 lemon
- 1 teaspoon dried thyme
- 1 teaspoon dried rosemary
- Salt and pepper to taste

Preparation:

1. In a bowl, mix olive oil, minced garlic, lemon zest, lemon juice, thyme, rosemary, salt, and pepper.
2. Place chicken breasts in the marinade and coat well. Give them at least half an hour to marinate.
3. Preheat grill to medium-high heat.
4. Grill chicken for 6-8 minutes per side until fully cooked.
5. Before serving, let it a few minutes to rest.

Portion Size: One serving (1 chicken breast)

Nutritional Information: Approximately 250 calories, 10g fat, 1g carbohydrates, 35g protein

4. Spaghetti Squash with Meatballs

Ingredients:

- 1 medium spaghetti squash
- 1-pound ground beef or turkey
- 1/4 cup almond flour (or breadcrumbs)
- 1 egg
- 1/4 cup grated Parmesan cheese
- 1 teaspoon Italian seasoning

- Marinara sauce
- Fresh basil for garnish

Preparation:

1. Preheat oven to 400°F (200°C).
2. Scoop out the seeds after cutting the spaghetti squash in half lengthwise.
3. Place the squash halves on a baking sheet, cut side down.
4. Bake for 40-50 minutes until the squash is tender. Scrape the strands with a folk.
5. In a bowl, mix ground meat, almond flour, egg, Parmesan, and Italian seasoning. Form into meatballs.
6. In a skillet, brown the meatballs on all sides.
7. Simmer meatballs in marinara sauce until cooked through.
8. Serve meatballs over spaghetti squash and garnish with fresh basil.

Portion Size: One serving

Nutritional Information: Approximately 300 calories, 15g fat, 15g carbohydrates, 25g protein

Ingredients:

- 1-pound beef sirloin, thinly sliced
- 2 cups broccoli florets
- 2 cloves garlic, minced
- 1 tablespoon sesame oil
- 2 tablespoons soy sauce (or tamari for low-carb)
- 1 tablespoon rice vinegar
- 1 teaspoon erythritol or preferred sweetener
- Salt, pepper, and red pepper flakes to taste

Preparation:

1. In a bowl, mix soy sauce, rice vinegar, sweetener, salt, pepper, and red pepper flakes. Set aside.
2. Heat sesame oil in a skillet or wok over high heat.
3. Add minced garlic and beef slices. Stir-fry until beef is browned.
4. Add broccoli florets and continue stir-frying for a few minutes until tender-crisp.
5. Pour the sauce mixture over the beef and broccoli.
6. Stir-fry for an additional minute until the sauce thickens.
7. Serve hot.

Portion Size: One serving

Nutritional Information: Approximately 280 calories, 15g fat, 8g carbohydrates, 30g protein

6. Stuffed Bell Peppers with Ground Turkey

Ingredients:

- Four bell peppers, cut in half, and seeds taken out.
- 1-pound ground turkey
- 1/2 cup cauliflower rice
- 1/4 cup diced onions
- 1/4 cup diced tomatoes
- 1/4 cup shredded cheese
- 1 teaspoon Italian seasoning
- Salt and pepper to taste

Preparation:

1. Preheat oven to 375°F (190°C).
2. Boil bell pepper halves in water for 5 minutes, then drain and set aside.
3. In a skillet, brown ground turkey with diced onions until cooked through.

4. Add cauliflower rice, diced tomatoes, Italian seasoning, salt, and pepper to the skillet. Cook for 5 minutes.
5. Spoon the turkey mixture into each bell pepper half.
6. Top with shredded cheese.
7. Bake for 20-25 minutes until the peppers are tender and cheese is melted.

Portion Size: One serving (2 pepper halves)

Nutritional Information: Approximately 280 calories, 15g fat, 10g carbohydrates, 25g protein

7. Eggplant Lasagna

Ingredients:

- 1 large eggplant, sliced lengthwise
- 1-pound ground beef or turkey
- 2 cups marinara sauce
- 1 cup ricotta cheese
- 1/2 cup shredded mozzarella cheese
- 1/4 cup grated Parmesan cheese
- Italian seasoning, salt, and pepper to taste

Preparation:

1. Preheat oven to 375°F (190°C).
2. Slice eggplant lengthwise into thin slices.
3. Grill or bake eggplant slices for 5-7 minutes until tender.
4. In a skillet, brown ground meat and season with Italian seasoning, salt, and pepper.
5. In a baking dish, layer marinara sauce, eggplant slices, ground meat, ricotta cheese, and repeat.
6. Top with shredded mozzarella and grated Parmesan cheese.
7. Cover with foil and bake for 25-30 minutes.
8. Remove foil and bake for an additional 10 minutes until cheese is golden and bubbly.

Portion Size: One serving

Nutritional Information: Approximately 320 calories, 20g fat, 10g carbohydrates, 25g protein

Ingredients:

- 4 chicken thighs (bone-in, skin-on)
- 2 tablespoons olive oil
- Zest and juice of 1 lemon
- 2 cloves garlic, minced
- 1 teaspoon dried thyme
- 1 teaspoon dried rosemary
- Garnish with Salt, pepper, and fresh parsley.

Preparation:

1. Preheat oven to 400°F (200°C).
2. In a bowl, mix olive oil, lemon zest, lemon juice, minced garlic, thyme, rosemary, salt, and pepper.
3. Place chicken thighs in a baking dish and coat with the lemon herb mixture.
4. Bake for 35-40 minutes until the chicken is cooked through and skin is crispy.
5. Garnish with fresh parsley before serving.

Portion Size: One serving (1 chicken thigh)

Nutritional Information: Approximately 280 calories, 20g fat, 1g carbohydrates, 25g protein

9. Shrimp Scampi with Zucchini Noodles

Ingredients:

- 1-pound shrimp, peeled and deveined
- 4 medium zucchinis (spiralized into noodles)
- 3 tablespoons butter
- 3 cloves garlic, minced
- Zest and juice of 1 lemon
- Red pepper flakes (optional)
- Salt, pepper, and fresh parsley for garnish

Preparation:

1. In a skillet, melt butter over medium heat.
2. Add minced garlic and red pepper flakes if using, sauté for 1-2 minutes.
3. Add shrimp and cook for 2-3 minutes per side until pink and opaque. Remove shrimp and set aside.
4. In the same skillet, add zucchini noodles, lemon zest, and lemon juice. Sauté for 2-3 minutes until tender.

5. Return cooked shrimp to the skillet and toss everything together.

6. Season with salt, pepper, and garnish with fresh parsley before serving.

Portion Size: One serving

Nutritional Information: Approximately 250 calories, 12g fat, 8g carbohydrates, 25g protein

10. Turkey Stuffed Portobello Mushrooms

Ingredients:

- 4 large Portobello mushrooms
- 1-pound ground turkey
- 1/2 cup diced onions
- 1/4 cup diced bell peppers
- 1/4 cup tomato sauce
- 1/4 cup shredded cheese
- Italian seasoning, salt, and pepper to taste
- Fresh basil for garnish

Preparation:

1. Preheat oven to 375°F (190°C).
2. Remove stems and gills from Portobello mushrooms.
3. In a skillet, brown ground turkey with diced onions and bell peppers.
4. Add tomato sauce, Italian seasoning, salt, and pepper to the skillet. Cook for 5 minutes.
5. Spoon turkey mixture into each mushroom cap.
6. Top with shredded cheese.
7. Bake for 20-25 minutes until mushrooms are tender and cheese is melted.
8. Garnish with fresh basil before serving.

Portion Size: One serving (1 stuffed mushroom)

Nutritional Information: Approximately 280 calories, 15g fat, 10g carbohydrates, 25g protein

Snack Recipes: Low-Carb Bites for Anytime Cravings:

1. Cucumber and Cream Cheese Bites

Ingredients:

- 1 cucumber, sliced into rounds
- 4 oz cream cheese
- One table spoon of freshly chopped parsley or dill.
- Salt and pepper to taste

Preparation:

1. In a bowl, mix cream cheese, chopped herbs, salt, and pepper.
2. Spread a small amount of the cream cheese mixture onto each cucumber slice.
3. Serve chilled.

Portion Size: One serving (5 cucumber rounds with cream cheese)

Nutritional Information: Approximately 80 calories, 7g fat, 2g carbohydrates, 2g protein

Ingredients:

- 6 hard-boiled eggs, peeled
- 2 tablespoons mayonnaise
- 1 teaspoon Dijon mustard
- Garnish with chopped parsley, chives, or paprika.
- Salt and pepper to taste

Preparation:

1. Slice the hard-boiled eggs in half lengthwise.
2. Scoop out the yolks into a bowl and mash them with mayonnaise, Dijon mustard, salt, and pepper.
3. Return the yolk mixture to the egg whites
4. Garnish with paprika, chopped chives, or parsley.

Portion Size: Three egg halves

Nutritional Information: Approximately 150 calories, 12g fat, 1g carbohydrates, 8g protein

Ingredients:

- 1 ripe avocado
- 1 can (5 oz) tuna, drained
- 1 tablespoon mayonnaise
- 1 tablespoon chopped red onion
- 1 tablespoon chopped cilantro
- Salt and pepper to taste

Preparation:

1. Cut the avocado in half and scoop out the flesh into a bowl, mashing it slightly.
2. Add drained tuna, mayonnaise, chopped red onion, cilantro, salt, and pepper to the bowl.
3. Mix everything until well combined.
4. Serve on lettuce leaves or cucumber slices.

Portion Size: One serving

Nutritional Information: Approximately 200 calories, 15g fat, 4g carbohydrates, 15g protein

Ingredients:

- 12 asparagus spears
- 6 slices bacon, halved lengthwise
- Olive oil for brushing (optional)
- Salt and pepper to taste

Preparation:

1. Preheat oven to 400°F (200°C) and line a baking sheet with parchment paper.
2. Wrap each asparagus spear with a half slice of bacon, starting from the bottom and spiraling to the top.
3. Place the wrapped asparagus on the baking sheet.
4. Optionally, brush with olive oil and season with salt and pepper.
5. Bake for 15-20 minutes until the bacon is crispy and asparagus is tender.

Portion Size: Three asparagus spears

Nutritional Information: Approximately 150 calories, 10g fat, 4g carbohydrates, 8g protein

Ingredients:

- One cup of shredded cheese, either mozzarella or cheddar, or to taste.
- Optional: seasoning (paprika, garlic powder, etc.)

Preparation:

1. Preheat oven to 350°F (175°C) and line a baking sheet with parchment paper.
2. Place small mounds of shredded cheese (about 1 tablespoon each) on the baking sheet, leaving space between each mound.
3. Optionally, sprinkle seasoning on top of each mound.
4. Bake for 5-7 minutes until the cheese crisps and edges turn golden.
5. Let them cool before removing from the baking sheet.

Portion Size: One serving (4-5 cheese crisps)

Nutritional Information: Approximately 120 calories, 10g fat, 1g carbohydrates, 7g protein

6. Zucchini Chips

Ingredients:

- 2 medium zucchinis, thinly sliced
- 2 tablespoons olive oil
- Salt, pepper, and garlic powder to taste

Preparation:

1. Preheat oven to 225°F (110°C) and line a baking sheet with parchment paper.
2. Place zucchini slices in a bowl and toss with olive oil, salt, pepper, and garlic powder until coated.
3. Arrange the slices on the baking sheet in a single layer.
4. Bake for 2-3 hours until the chips are crispy, flipping them halfway through.

Portion Size: One serving (about 10-12 chips)

Nutritional Information: Approximately 100 calories, 7g fat, 5g carbohydrates, 3g protein

6. Zucchini Chips

Ingredients:

- 12 slices pepperoni
- 2 oz sliced cheese (cheddar, mozzarella, or your choice)

Preparation:

1. Place a slice of cheese on each pepperoni slice.
2. Roll them up tightly and secure with a toothpick if needed.
3. Serve as is or lightly heat in the microwave for a melty snack.

Portion Size: One serving (3 roll-ups)

Nutritional Information: Approximately 150 calories, 12g fat, 1g carbohydrates, 9g protein

Ingredients:

- 1 cup Greek yogurt (unsweetened)
- 1/4 cup of fresh raspberries, blue berries, and strawberries.
- 1 tablespoon chopped nuts or seeds
- Optional: a drizzle of sugar-free sweetener

Preparation:

1. Arrange fresh berries and Greek yoghurt in a bowl or glass.
2. Sprinkle chopped nuts or seeds on top.
3. Optionally, drizzle with a sugar-free sweetener for added sweetness.

Portion Size: One serving

Nutritional Information: Approximately 150 calories, 5g fat, 10g carbohydrates, 15g protein

Ingredients:

- Cherry tomatoes
- Fresh mozzarella balls (bocconcini)
- Fresh basil leaves
- Balsamic glaze for drizzling (optional)

Preparation:

1. Skewer a cherry tomato, a small mozzarella ball, and a basil leaf onto toothpicks or small skewers.
2. Arrange the skewers on a serving plate.
3. Optionally, drizzle with balsamic glaze before serving.

Portion Size: One serving (3-4 skewers)

Nutritional Information: Approximately 100 calories, 6g fat, 3g carbohydrates, 6g protein

Ingredients:

- 2 celery stalks, cut into sticks
- 2 tablespoons almond butter

Preparation:

1. Spread almond butter onto celery sticks.
2. Serve as a crunchy and satisfying snack.

Portion Size: One serving

Nutritional Information: Approximately 150 calories, 12g fat, 6g carbohydrates, 6g protein

Dessert Recipes: Indulgent Low-Carb Treats:

1. Chocolate Avocado Mousse

Ingredients:

- 2 ripe avocados
- 1/4 cup unsweetened cocoa powder
- 1/4 cup low-carb sweetener (such as erythritol or stevia)
- 1 teaspoon vanilla extract
- Pinch of salt
- Optional: whipped cream and berries for garnish

Preparation:

1. In a food processor or blender, combine avocados, cocoa powder, sweetener, vanilla extract, and salt.
2. Blend until smooth and creamy.
3. Spoon into serving dishes and chill for at least 30 minutes.
4. Garnish with whipped cream and berries if desired.

Portion Size: One serving

Nutritional Information: Approximately 200 calories, 15g fat, 10g carbohydrates, 5g protein

2. Low-Carb Cheesecake Bars

Ingredients:

- 2 cups almond flour
- 1/4 cup low-carb sweetener
- 1/2 cup butter, melted
- 16 oz cream cheese, softened
- 2 eggs
- 1 teaspoon vanilla extract
- Optional: sugar-free fruit topping

Preparation:

1. Preheat oven to 350°F (175°C) and line a baking dish with parchment paper.
2. In a bowl, combine almond flour, sweetener, and melted butter to form the crust mixture.
3. Press the crust mixture evenly into the bottom of the baking dish.
4. In another bowl, beat cream cheese, eggs, sweetener, and vanilla extract until smooth.

5. Pour the cream cheese mixture over the crust.

6. Bake for 25-30 minutes until the edges are set but the center is slightly jiggly.

7. Let it cool, then refrigerate for at least 2 hours before slicing into bars.

8. Top with sugar-free fruit topping if desired.

Portion Size: One bar

Nutritional Information: Approximately 200 calories, 18g fat, 4g carbohydrates, 6g protein

3. Keto Peanut Butter Cookies

Ingredients:

- 1 cup peanut butter (sugar-free)
- 1/2 cup low-carb sweetener
- 1 egg

Preparation:

1. Preheat oven to 350°F (175°C) and line a baking sheet with parchment paper.

2. In a bowl, mix peanut butter, sweetener, and egg until well combined.

3. Roll the dough into small balls and place them on the baking sheet.

4. Use a fork to flatten each cookie and create a crisscross pattern.

5. Bake for 10-12 minutes until the edges are golden.

6. Let the cookies cool on the baking sheet before serving.

Portion Size: One cookie

Nutritional Information: Approximately 120 calories, 10g fat, 3g carbohydrates, 5g protein

4. Coconut Flour Chocolate Chip Cookies

Ingredients:

- 1/2 cup coconut flour
- 1/2 cup butter, softened
- 1/3 cup low-carb sweetener
- 2 eggs
- 1 teaspoon vanilla extract
- 1/4 cup sugar-free chocolate chips

Preparation:

1. Preheat oven to 350°F (175°C) and line a baking sheet with parchment paper.
2. In a bowl, cream together butter and sweetener.
3. Add eggs and vanilla extract, and mix well.
4. Gradually add coconut flour and mix until combined.
5. Fold in sugar-free chocolate chips.
6. Form the dough into small balls, place them on the baking sheet, and flatten slightly.
7. Bake for 12-15 minutes until the edges are golden.
8. Let the cookies cool before serving.

Portion Size: One cookie

Nutritional Information: Approximately 90 calories, 7g fat, 3g carbohydrates, 2g protein

Ingredients:

- 1 cup shredded unsweetened coconut
- 1/4 cup coconut oil, melted
- 2 tablespoons low-carb sweetener
- Zest and juice of 1 lemon

Preparation:

1. In a bowl, combine shredded coconut, melted coconut oil, sweetener, lemon zest, and lemon juice.
2. Mix until well combined and the mixture holds together.
3. Roll the mixture into small balls and place them on a plate.
4. Refrigerate for at least 30 minutes before serving.

Portion Size: Two balls

Nutritional Information: Approximately 120 calories, 12g fat, 2g carbohydrates, 1g protein

Ingredients:

- 2 cups heavy cream
- 1/4 cup low-carb sweetener
- 1 teaspoon vanilla extract
- 2 tablespoons gelatin powder
- 1 cup of mixed berries, either frozen or fresh.

Preparation:

1. In a saucepan, heat heavy cream and sweetener over medium heat, stirring until sweetener dissolves.
2. After taking off the heat, whisk in the vanilla essence.
3. Sprinkle gelatin powder over the cream mixture and whisk until dissolved.
4. Divide the mixture among serving glasses or molds.
5. Chill in the refrigerator for at least 4 hours until set.
6. Top with mixed berries before serving.

Portion Size: One serving

Nutritional Information: Approximately 250 calories, 25g fat, 5g carbohydrates, 3g protein

Ingredients:

- 1 cup sugar-free dark chocolate chips
- 12 large strawberries, washed and dried

Preparation:

1. Use parchment paper to line a baking sheet.
2. In a microwave-safe bowl, melt the dark chocolate chips in 30-second intervals, stirring in between until smooth.
3. Dip each strawberry into the melted chocolate, coating them halfway.
4. Place the dipped strawberries on the prepared baking sheet.
5. Refrigerate until the chocolate sets.

Portion Size: Three strawberries

Nutritional Information: Approximately 150 calories, 10g fat, 10g carbohydrates, 2g protein

Ingredients:

- 1 1/2 cups almond flour
- 1/2 cup low-carb sweetener
- Zest and juice of 2 lemons
- 1/4 cup melted butter
- 3 eggs
- 1 teaspoon baking powder
- Pinch of salt

Preparation:

1. Warm up the oven to 350°F (175°C) and coat a cake pan with oil.
2. In a bowl, mix almond flour, sweetener, lemon zest, melted butter, eggs, baking powder, lemon juice, and salt until smooth.
3. Pour the batter into the cake pan and smooth the top.
4. Bake for 25-30 minutes until a toothpick inserted in the center comes out clean.
5. Let the cake cool before slicing.

Portion Size: One slice

Nutritional Information: Approximately 200 calories, 18g fat, 5g carbohydrates, 6g protein

9. Keto-Friendly Vanilla Ice Cream

Ingredients:

- 2 cups heavy cream
- 1 cup almond milk (unsweetened)
- 1/2 cup low-carb sweetener
- 2 teaspoons vanilla extract

Preparation:

1. In a bowl, mix heavy cream, almond milk, sweetener, and vanilla extract until well combined.
2. Pour the mixture into an ice cream maker and churn according to the manufacturer's instructions.
3. Transfer the churned ice cream to a freezer-safe container and freeze for at least 4 hours before serving.

Portion Size: One serving

Nutritional Information: Approximately 250 calories, 25g fat, 5g carbohydrates, 2g protein

Ingredients:

- 2 cups almond flour
- 1/4 cup low-carb sweetener
- 1 teaspoon baking powder
- 1 teaspoon pumpkin pie spice
- 1/2 cup pumpkin puree
- 1/4 cup melted butter
- 2 eggs
- 1 teaspoon vanilla extract

Preparation:

1. Preheat oven to 350°F (175°C) and line a muffin tin with liners.
2. In a bowl, whisk together almond flour, sweetener, baking powder, and pumpkin pie spice.
3. In another bowl, mix pumpkin puree, melted butter, eggs, and vanilla extract.
4. Combine the wet and dry ingredients until well incorporated.
5. Divide the batter into the muffin cups.

6. Bake for 20-25 minutes until a toothpick inserted in the center comes out clean.

7. Let the muffins cool before serving.

Portion Size: One muffin

Nutritional Information: Approximately 180 calories, 15g fat, 5g carbohydrates, 6g protein

30-DAY MEAL PLAN

DAY 1

BREAKFAST: Spinach and Feta Omelette

LUNCH: Tuna Stuffed Bell Peppers

DINNER: Lemon Garlic Butter Salmon

SNACK: Almond Butter Celery Sticks

DESSERT: Chocolate Avocado Mousse

DAY 2

BREAKFAST: Greek Yogurt Parfait

LUNCH: Keto Chicken Cobb Salad

DINNER: Cauliflower Crust Pizza

SNACK: Mini Caprese Skewers

DESSERT: Low-Carb Cheesecake Bars

DAY 3

BREAKFAST: Avocado and Bacon Breakfast Bowl

LUNCH: Chicken and Avocado Salad

DINNER: Grilled Lemon Herb Chicken

SNACK: Greek Yogurt Parfait

DESSERT: Keto Peanut Butter Cookies

DAY 4

BREAKFAST: Coconut Flour Pancakes

LUNCH: Low-Carb Turkey Taco Lettuce Cups

DINNER: Spaghetti Squash with Meatballs

SNACK: Pepperoni and Cheese Roll-Ups

DESSERT: Coconut Flour Chocolate Chip Cookies

DAY 5

BREAKFAST: Smoked Salmon and Cream Cheese Roll-ups

LUNCH: Egg Salad Lettuce Wraps

DINNER: Stir-Fried Beef and Broccoli

SNACK: Zucchini Chips

DESSERT: Lemon Coconut Balls

DAY 6

BREAKFAST: Zucchini and Cheese Frittata Muffins

LUNCH: Greek Salad with Grilled Halloumi

DINNER: Stuffed Bell Peppers with Ground Turkey

SNACK: Cheese Crisps

DESSERT: Sugar-Free Berry Panna Cotta

DAY 7

BREAKFAST: Cauliflower Hash Browns

LUNCH: Cauliflower Fried Rice with Shrimp

DINNER: Eggplant Lasagna

SNACK: Bacon-Wrapped Asparagus

DESSERT: Dark Chocolate Dipped Strawberries

DAY 8

BREAKFAST: Turkey and Cheese Breakfast Roll-ups

LUNCH: Turkey Lettuce Wraps

DINNER: Baked Lemon Herb Chicken Thighs

SNACK: Avocado Tuna Salad

DESSERT: Almond Flour Lemon Cake

DAY 9

BREAKFAST: Chia Seed Pudding

LUNCH: Zucchini Noodles with Pesto and Cherry Tomatoes

DINNER: Shrimp Scampi with Zucchini Noodles

SNACK: Deviled Eggs

DESSERT: Keto-Friendly Vanilla Ice Cream

DAY 10

BREAKFAST: Keto Green Smoothie

LUNCH: Grilled Chicken Caesar Salad

DINNER: Turkey Stuffed Portobello Mushrooms

SNACK: Cucumber and Cream Cheese Bites

DESSERT: Sugar-Free Pumpkin Spice Muffins

DAY 11

BREAKFAST: Spinach and Feta Omelette

LUNCH: Tuna Stuffed Bell Peppers

DINNER: Lemon Garlic Butter Salmon

SNACK: Almond Butter Celery Sticks

DESSERT: Chocolate Avocado Mousse

DAY 12

BREAKFAST: Greek Yogurt Parfait

LUNCH: Keto Chicken Cobb Salad

DINNER: Cauliflower Crust Pizza

SNACK: Mini Caprese Skewers

DESSERT: Low-Carb Cheesecake Bars

DAY 13

BREAKFAST: Avocado and Bacon Breakfast Bowl

LUNCH: Chicken and Avocado Salad

DINNER: Grilled Lemon Herb Chicken

SNACK: Greek Yogurt Parfait

DESSERT: Keto Peanut Butter Cookies

DAY 14

BREAKFAST: Coconut Flour Pancakes

LUNCH: Low-Carb Turkey Taco Lettuce Cups

DINNER: Spaghetti Squash with Meatballs

SNACK: Pepperoni and Cheese Roll-Ups

DESSERT: Coconut Flour Chocolate Chip Cookies

DAY 15

BREAKFAST: Smoked Salmon and Cream Cheese Roll-ups

LUNCH: Egg Salad Lettuce Wraps

DINNER: Stir-Fried Beef and Broccoli

SNACK: Zucchini Chips

DESSERT: Lemon Coconut Balls

DAY 16

BREAKFAST: Zucchini and Cheese Frittata Muffins

LUNCH: Greek Salad with Grilled Halloumi

DINNER: Stuffed Bell Peppers with Ground Turkey

SNACK: Cheese Crisps

DESSERT: Sugar-Free Berry Panna Cotta

DAY 17

BREAKFAST: Cauliflower Hash Browns

LUNCH: Cauliflower Fried Rice with Shrimp

DINNER: Eggplant Lasagna

SNACK: Bacon-Wrapped Asparagus

DESSERT: Dark Chocolate Dipped Strawberries

DAY 18

BREAKFAST: Turkey and Cheese Breakfast Roll-ups

LUNCH: Turkey Lettuce Wraps

DINNER: Baked Lemon Herb Chicken Thighs

SNACK: Avocado Tuna Salad

DESSERT: Almond Flour Lemon Cake

DAY 19

BREAKFAST: Chia Seed Pudding

LUNCH: Zucchini Noodles with Pesto and Cherry Tomatoes

DINNER: Shrimp Scampi with Zucchini Noodles

SNACK: Deviled Eggs

DESSERT: Keto-Friendly Vanilla Ice Cream

DAY 20

BREAKFAST: Keto Green Smoothie

LUNCH: Grilled Chicken Caesar Salad

DINNER: Turkey Stuffed Portobello Mushrooms

SNACK: Cucumber and Cream Cheese Bites

DESSERT: Sugar-Free Pumpkin Spice Muffins

DAY 21

BREAKFAST: Spinach and Feta Omelette

LUNCH: Tuna Stuffed Bell Peppers

DINNER: Lemon Garlic Butter Salmon

SNACK: Almond Butter Celery Sticks

DESSERT: Chocolate Avocado Mousse

DAY 22

BREAKFAST: Greek Yogurt Parfait

LUNCH: Keto Chicken Cobb Salad

DINNER: Cauliflower Crust Pizza

SNACK: Mini Caprese Skewers

DESSERT: Low-Carb Cheesecake Bars

DAY 23

BREAKFAST: Avocado and Bacon Breakfast Bowl

LUNCH: Chicken and Avocado Salad

DINNER: Grilled Lemon Herb Chicken

SNACK: Greek Yogurt Parfait

DESSERT: Keto Peanut Butter Cookies

DAY 24

BREAKFAST: Coconut Flour Pancakes

LUNCH: Low-Carb Turkey Taco Lettuce Cups

DINNER: Spaghetti Squash with Meatballs

SNACK: Pepperoni and Cheese Roll-Ups

DESSERT: Coconut Flour Chocolate Chip Cookies

DAY 25

BREAKFAST: Smoked Salmon and Cream Cheese Roll-ups

LUNCH: Egg Salad Lettuce Wraps

DINNER: Stir-Fried Beef and Broccoli

SNACK: Zucchini Chips

DESSERT: Lemon Coconut Balls

DAY 26

BREAKFAST: Zucchini and Cheese Frittata Muffins

LUNCH: Greek Salad with Grilled Halloumi

DINNER: Stuffed Bell Peppers with Ground Turkey

SNACK: Cheese Crisps

DESSERT: Sugar-Free Berry Panna Cotta

DAY 27

BREAKFAST: Cauliflower Hash Browns

LUNCH: Cauliflower Fried Rice with Shrimp

DINNER: Eggplant Lasagna

SNACK: Bacon-Wrapped Asparagus

DESSERT: Dark Chocolate Dipped Strawberries

DAY 28

BREAKFAST: Turkey and Cheese Breakfast Roll-ups

LUNCH: Turkey Lettuce Wraps

DINNER: Baked Lemon Herb Chicken Thighs

SNACK: Avocado Tuna Salad

DESSERT: Almond Flour Lemon Cake

DAY 29

BREAKFAST: Chia Seed Pudding

LUNCH: Zucchini Noodles with Pesto and Cherry Tomatoes

DINNER: Shrimp Scampi with Zucchini Noodles

SNACK: Deviled Eggs

DESSERT: Keto-Friendly Vanilla Ice Cream

DAY 30

BREAKFAST: Keto Green Smoothie

LUNCH: Grilled Chicken Caesar Salad

DINNER: Turkey Stuffed Portobello Mushrooms

SNACK: Cucumber and Cream Cheese Bites

DESSERT: Sugar-Free Pumpkin Spice Muffins

To enhance success on this dietary plan, several key aspects play crucial roles, encompassing exercise and physical activity guidelines, strategies to overcome challenges and stay motivated, and addressing common questions and troubleshooting issues.

Exercise and Physical Activity Guidelines:

Physical activity is a vital component of a healthy lifestyle, complementing the Atkins Diet's principles. Incorporating exercise can amplify the diet's effectiveness and overall well-being. The Atkins Diet encourages moderate physical activity aligned with an individual's fitness level. Here's a guideline to enhance success:

Cardiovascular Exercise: Engaging in activities like brisk walking, cycling, swimming, or jogging for 30-60 minutes most days of the week can boost metabolism and aid in weight management.

Strength Training: Adding strength training exercises, using body weight or resistance bands, helps build muscle, which supports metabolic health and burns more calories even at rest.

Flexibility and Balance: Integrating stretching, yoga, or Pilates enhances flexibility, posture, and balance, supporting overall fitness and reducing injury risk.

Consistency and Progression: Gradually increase exercise duration and intensity, aiming for a mix of aerobic and strength exercises for a well-rounded routine.

Overcoming Challenges and Staying Motivated:

Meal Planning and Preparation: Plan meals in advance, ensuring access to low-carb, Atkins-friendly options to avoid impulsive, high-carb choices. Batch cooking and storing meals can simplify adherence.

Social Situations: Navigate social gatherings by communicating dietary preferences to hosts and bringing Atkins-friendly dishes. Give socializing more attention than just eating.

Cravings and Temptations: Combat cravings by having low-carb snacks readily available. Opt for healthy fats, proteins, and fiber-rich foods to keep hunger and cravings at bay.

Tracking Progress: Monitor changes in weight, measurements, and overall well-being to stay motivated. Celebrate small milestones and acknowledge progress.

Mindset and Support: Cultivate a positive mindset, focusing on health improvements rather than just weight loss. Ask for help and guidance from friends, family, and internet networks.

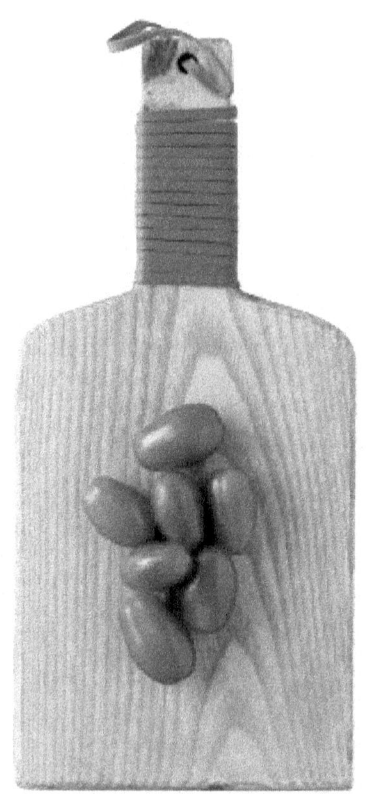

CONCLUSION

Embracing the Atkins Diet entails a comprehensive commitment to health and well-being. By intertwining dietary adjustments with exercise guidelines, strategies to surmount challenges, and addressing common queries, individuals can navigate this journey with confidence.

Exercise forms a pivotal component, synergizing with the Atkins Diet to optimize results. Incorporating cardiovascular, strength, flexibility, and balance exercises, tailored to individual capabilities, magnifies the diet's efficacy and fosters holistic wellness.

Overcoming hurdles and sustaining motivation are intrinsic to success. Planning meals, navigating social settings, managing cravings, and celebrating progress fortify the journey. Cultivating a positive mindset and seeking support embolden individuals, fostering resilience amidst challenges.

Addressing frequently asked questions and troubleshooting common issues empowers individuals with insights and solutions.

From plateauing weight loss to digestive concerns, proactive measures, including dietary adjustments and professional consultation, pave the way forward.

Ultimately, the Atkins Diet transcends mere dietary modification; it champions a lifestyle shift. Embracing exercise, conquering obstacles, and seeking solutions converge to sculpt a path towards sustainable health improvements. Each step, each triumph, contributes to a tapestry of wellness woven with dedication and perseverance.

In this holistic approach, the Atkins Diet thrives, not just as a dietary regimen, but as a compass guiding individual towards enduring vitality and balanced living. By embracing this journey with resilience, adaptability, and determination, individuals can unravel the true potential of the Atkins Diet, achieving lasting health and well-being.

WEEKLY MEAL JOURNAL

WEEK ___________________ MONTH ___________________

MONDAY

SATURDAY

TUESDAY

SUNDAY

WEDNESDAY

SHOPPING LIST

THURSDAY

FRIDAY

NOTES:

WEEKLY
MEAL JOURNAL

WEEK ___________________   MONTH ___________________

MONDAY

SATURDAY

TUESDAY

SUNDAY

WEDNESDAY

SHOPPING LIST

THURSDAY

FRIDAY

NOTES:

WEEKLY
MEAL JOURNAL

WEEK ___________________   MONTH ___________________

MONDAY

SATURDAY

TUESDAY

SUNDAY

WEDNESDAY

SHOPPING LIST

THURSDAY

FRIDAY

NOTES:

WEEKLY
MEAL JOURNAL

WEEK _______________ MONTH _______________

MONDAY

SATURDAY

TUESDAY

SUNDAY

WEDNESDAY

SHOPPING LIST

THURSDAY

FRIDAY

NOTES:

WEEKLY
MEAL JOURNAL

WEEK _______________   MONTH _______________

MONDAY

SATURDAY

TUESDAY

SUNDAY

WEDNESDAY

SHOPPING LIST

THURSDAY

FRIDAY

NOTES:

WEEKLY
MEAL JOURNAL

WEEK _______________   MONTH _______________

MONDAY

SATURDAY

TUESDAY

SUNDAY

WEDNESDAY

SHOPPING LIST

THURSDAY

FRIDAY

NOTES:

WEEKLY MEAL JOURNAL

WEEK ________________ MONTH ________________

MONDAY

TUESDAY

WEDNESDAY

THURSDAY

FRIDAY

SATURDAY

SUNDAY

SHOPPING LIST

- ○ _______________
- ○ _______________
- ○ _______________
- ○ _______________
- ○ _______________
- ○ _______________
- ○ _______________
- ○ _______________

NOTES:

- ○ _______________
- ○ _______________
- ○ _______________
- ○ _______________

WEEKLY
MEAL JOURNAL

WEEK ________________________   MONTH ________________________

MONDAY	SATURDAY

TUESDAY	SUNDAY

WEDNESDAY

THURSDAY

FRIDAY

SHOPPING LIST

- ____________________
- ____________________
- ____________________
- ____________________
- ____________________
- ____________________
- ____________________
- ____________________

NOTES:

- ____________________
- ____________________
- ____________________
- ____________________

WEEKLY
MEAL JOURNAL

WEEK ___________________   MONTH ___________________

MONDAY

SATURDAY

TUESDAY

SUNDAY

WEDNESDAY

SHOPPING LIST

○ _______________________
○ _______________________
○ _______________________
○ _______________________
○ _______________________
○ _______________________
○ _______________________
○ _______________________

THURSDAY

FRIDAY

NOTES:

○ _______________________
○ _______________________
○ _______________________
○ _______________________

WEEKLY
MEAL JOURNAL

WEEK _______________________   MONTH _______________________

MONDAY

SATURDAY

TUESDAY

SUNDAY

WEDNESDAY

SHOPPING LIST

○ _______________________
○ _______________________
○ _______________________
○ _______________________
○ _______________________
○ _______________________
○ _______________________
○ _______________________

THURSDAY

FRIDAY

○ NOTES:
○ _______________________
○ _______________________
○ _______________________

WEEKLY
MEAL JOURNAL

WEEK _______________ MONTH _______________

MONDAY

TUESDAY

WEDNESDAY

THURSDAY

FRIDAY

SATURDAY

SUNDAY

SHOPPING LIST

- ________________
- ________________
- ________________
- ________________
- ________________
- ________________
- ________________
- ________________

NOTES:

- ________________
- ________________
- ________________
- ________________

WEEKLY MEAL JOURNAL

WEEK ______________________   MONTH ______________________

MONDAY

TUESDAY

WEDNESDAY

THURSDAY

FRIDAY

SATURDAY

SUNDAY

SHOPPING LIST

○ ______________________
○ ______________________
○ ______________________
○ ______________________
○ ______________________
○ ______________________
○ ______________________
○ ______________________

NOTES:

○ ______________________
○ ______________________
○ ______________________
○ ______________________